For More Information

This booklet is only one of many free booklets for people with cancer. Here are some others you may find useful:

- *Biological Therapy*
- *Chemotherapy and You: Support for People With Cancer*
- *Eating Hints: Before, During, and After Cancer Treatment*
- *Taking Part in Cancer Treatment Research Studies*
- *Thinking About Complementary & Alternative Medicine: A Guide for People With Cancer*
- *Pain Control: Support for People With Cancer*
- *When Cancer Returns*
- *Taking Time: Support for People With Cancer*

These booklets are available from the National Cancer Institute (often called NCI). NCI is a federal agency that is part of the National Institutes of Health. Call 1-800-4-CANCER (1-800-422-6237) or visit www.cancer.gov. (See page 59 for more information.)

*For information about your specific type of cancer, see the PDQ® database. PDQ® is NCI's complete cancer database. You can find it at www.cancer.gov.

Product or brand names that appear in this book are for example only. The U.S. Government does not endorse any specific product or brand. If products or brands are not mentioned, it does not mean or imply that they are not satisfactory.

1-800-4-CANCER (1-800-422-6237)

About This Book

Radiation Therapy and You is written for you—someone who is about to get or is now getting radiation therapy for cancer. People who are close to you may also find this book helpful.

This book is a guide that you can refer to throughout radiation therapy. It has facts about radiation therapy and side effects and describes how you can care for yourself during and after treatment.

> Rather than read this book from beginning to end— <u>look at only those sections you need now.</u> Later, you can always read more.

This book covers:

- **Questions and Answers About Radiation Therapy.** Answers to common questions, such as what radiation therapy is and how it affects cancer cells.

- **External Beam and Internal Radiation.** Information about the two types of radiation therapy.

- **Your Feelings During Radiation Therapy.** Information about feelings, such as depression and anxiety, and ways to cope with them.

- **Side Effects and Ways To Manage Them.** A chart that shows problems that may happen as a result of treatment and ways you can help manage them.

- **Questions To Ask.** Questions for you to think about and discuss with your doctor, nurse, and others involved in your treatment and care.

- **Lists of Foods and Liquids.** Foods and drinks you can have during radiation therapy.

- **Words To Know.** A dictionary that clearly explains medical terms used in this book. These terms are in bold print the first time they appear.

- **Ways To Learn More.** Places to go for more information—in print, online (Internet), and by telephone.

Talk with your doctor and nurse about the information in this book. They may suggest that you read certain sections or follow some of the tips. Since radiation therapy affects people in different ways, they may also tell you that some of the information in this book is not right for you.

www.cancer.gov

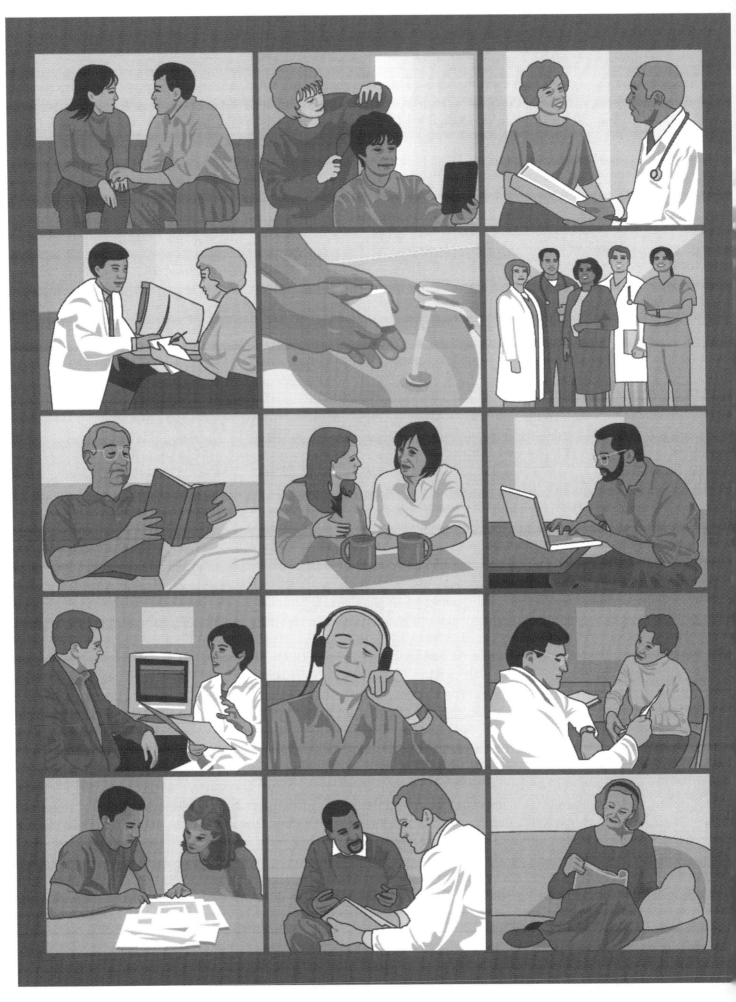

Table of Contents

Questions and Answers About Radiation Therapy 1

External Beam Radiation Therapy 9

Internal Radiation Therapy 15

Your Feelings During Radiation Therapy 19

Radiation Therapy Side Effects 21
- Radiation Therapy Side Effects At-A-Glance 23
- Radiation Therapy Side Effects and Ways to Manage Them 24
  - Diarrhea 24
  - Fatigue 26
  - Hair Loss 28
  - Mouth Changes 30
  - Nausea and Vomiting 34
  - Sexual and Fertility Changes 36
  - Skin Changes 40
  - Throat Changes 43
  - Urinary and Bladder Changes 45
- Late Radiation Therapy Side Effects 47

Questions To Ask Your Doctor or Nurse 51

Lists of Foods and Liquids 53
- Clear Liquids 53
- Foods and Drinks That Are High in Calories or Protein 54
- Foods and Drinks That Are Easy on the Stomach 55

Words To Know 56

Resources for Learning More 59

> Rather than read this book from beginning to end— *look at only those sections you need now.* Later, you can always read more.

www.cancer.gov

Questions and Answers About Radiation Therapy

What is radiation therapy?

Radiation therapy (also called **radiotherapy**) is a cancer treatment that uses high doses of radiation to kill cancer cells and stop them from spreading. At low doses, radiation is used as an x-ray to see inside your body and take pictures, such as x-rays of your teeth or broken bones. Radiation used in cancer treatment works in much the same way, except that it is given at higher doses.

How is radiation therapy given?

Radiation therapy can be **external beam** (when a machine outside your body aims radiation at cancer cells) or **internal** (when radiation is put inside your body, in or near the cancer cells). Sometimes people get both forms of radiation therapy. To learn more about external beam radiation therapy, see page 9. To learn more about internal radiation therapy, see page 15.

Who gets radiation therapy?

Many people with cancer need radiation therapy. In fact, more than half (about 60 percent) of people with cancer get radiation therapy. Sometimes, radiation therapy is the only kind of cancer treatment people need.

What does radiation therapy do to cancer cells?

Given in high doses, radiation kills or slows the growth of cancer cells. Radiation therapy is used to:

- **Treat cancer.** Radiation can be used to cure, stop, or slow the growth of cancer.

- **Reduce symptoms.** When a cure is not possible, radiation may be used to shrink cancer tumors in order to reduce pressure. Radiation therapy used in this way can treat problems such as pain, or it can prevent problems such as blindness or loss of bowel and bladder control.

www.cancer.gov

How long does radiation therapy take to work?

Radiation therapy does not kill cancer cells right away. It takes days or weeks of treatment before cancer cells start to die. Then, cancer cells keep dying for weeks or months after radiation therapy ends.

What does radiation therapy do to healthy cells?

Radiation not only kills or slows the growth of cancer cells, it can also affect nearby healthy cells. The healthy cells almost always recover after treatment is over. But sometimes people may have side effects that do not get better or are severe. Doctors try to protect healthy cells during treatment by:

- **Using as low a dose of radiation as possible.** The radiation dose is balanced between being high enough to kill cancer cells yet low enough to limit damage to healthy cells.

- **Spreading out treatment over time.** You may get radiation therapy once a day for several weeks or in smaller doses twice a day. Spreading out the radiation dose allows normal cells to recover while cancer cells die.

- **Aiming radiation at a precise part of your body.** New techniques, such as **IMRT** and **3-D conformal radiation therapy,** allow your doctor to aim higher doses of radiation at your cancer while reducing the radiation to nearby healthy tissue.

- **Using medicines.** Some drugs can help protect certain parts of your body, such as the salivary glands that make saliva (spit).

Does radiation therapy hurt?

No, radiation therapy does not hurt while it is being given. But the side effects that people may get from radiation therapy can cause pain or discomfort. This book has a lot of information about ways that you, your doctor, and your nurse can help manage side effects.

Is radiation therapy used with other types of cancer treatment?

Yes, radiation therapy is often used with other cancer treatments. Here are some examples:

- **Radiation therapy and surgery.** Radiation may be given before, during, or after surgery. Doctors may use radiation to shrink the size of the cancer before surgery, or they may use radiation after surgery to kill any cancer cells that remain. Sometimes, radiation therapy is given during surgery so that it goes straight to the cancer without passing through the skin. This is called intraoperative radiation.

- **Radiation therapy and chemotherapy.** Radiation may be given before, during, or after chemotherapy. Before or during chemotherapy, radiation therapy can shrink the cancer so that chemotherapy works better. Sometimes, chemotherapy is given to help radiation therapy work better. After chemotherapy, radiation therapy can be used to kill any cancer cells that remain.

Who is on my radiation therapy team?

Many people help with your radiation treatment and care. This group of health care providers is often called the "radiation therapy team." They work together to provide care that is just right for you. Your radiation therapy team can include:

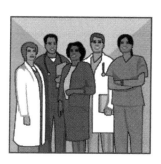

- **Radiation oncologist.** This is a doctor who specializes in using radiation therapy to treat cancer. He or she prescribes how much radiation you will receive, plans how your treatment will be given, closely follows you during your course of treatment, and prescribes care you may need to help with side effects. He or she works closely with the other doctors, nurses, and health care providers on your team. After you are finished with radiation therapy, your radiation oncologist will see you for follow-up visits. During these visits, this doctor will check for **late side effects** and assess how well the radiation has worked.

- **Nurse practitioner.** This is a nurse with advanced training. He or she can take your medical history, do physical exams, order tests, manage side effects, and closely watch your response to treatment. After you are finished with radiation therapy, your nurse practitioner may see you for follow-up visits to check for late side effects and assess how well the radiation has worked.

www.cancer.gov

You are the most important part of the radiation therapy team.

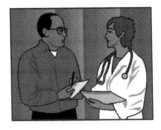

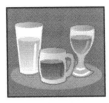

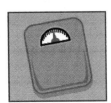

- **Radiation nurse.** This person provides nursing care during radiation therapy, working with all the members of your radiation therapy team. He or she will talk with you about your radiation treatment and help you manage side effects.

- **Radiation therapist.** This person works with you during each radiation therapy session. He or she positions you for treatment and runs the machines to make sure you get the dose of radiation prescribed by your radiation oncologist.

- **Other health care providers.** Your team may also include a dietitian, physical therapist, social worker, and others.

- **You.** You are also part of the radiation therapy team. Your role is to:
  - Arrive on time for all radiation therapy sessions
  - Ask questions and talk about your concerns
  - Let someone on your radiation therapy team know when you have side effects
  - Tell your doctor or nurse if you are in pain
  - Follow the advice of your doctors and nurses about how to care for yourself at home, such as:
    - Taking care of your skin
    - Drinking liquids
    - Eating foods that they suggest
    - Keeping your weight the same

Be sure to arrive on time for ALL radiation therapy sessions.

Is radiation therapy expensive?

Yes, radiation therapy costs a lot of money. It uses complex machines and involves the services of many health care providers. The exact cost of your radiation therapy depends on the cost of health care where you live, what kind of radiation therapy you get, and how many treatments you need.

Talk with your health insurance company about what services it will pay for. Most insurance plans pay for radiation therapy for their members. To learn more, talk with the business office where you get treatment. You can also contact the National Cancer Institute's Cancer Information Service and ask for the "Financial Assistance for Cancer Care" fact sheet. See page 59 for ways to contact the National Cancer Institute.

Should I follow a special diet while I am getting radiation therapy?

Your body uses a lot of energy to heal during radiation therapy. It is important that you eat enough calories and protein to keep your weight the same during this time. Ask your doctor or nurse if you need a special diet while you are getting radiation therapy. You might also find it helpful to speak with a dietitian.

To learn more about foods and drinks that are high in calories or protein, see the chart on page 54. You may also want to read Eating Hints, a book from the National Cancer Institute. You can order a free copy online at http://www.cancer.gov/publications or 1-800-4-CANCER.

> *Ask your doctor, nurse, or dietitian if you need a special diet while you are getting radiation therapy.*

Can I go to work during radiation therapy?

Some people are able to work full-time during radiation therapy. Others can only work part-time or not at all. How much you are able to work depends on how you feel. Ask your doctor or nurse what you may expect based on the treatment you are getting.

You are likely to feel well enough to work when you start radiation therapy. As time goes on, do not be surprised if you are more tired, have less energy, or feel weak. Once you have finished your treatment, it may take a few weeks or many months for you to feel better.

You may get to a point during your radiation therapy when you feel too sick to work. Talk with your employer to find out if you can go on **medical leave**. Make sure that your health insurance will pay for treatment when you are on medical leave.

What happens when radiation therapy is over?

Once you have finished radiation therapy, you will need **follow-up care** for the rest of your life. Follow-up care refers to checkups with your radiation oncologist or nurse practitioner after your course of radiation therapy is over. During these checkups, your doctor or nurse will see how well the radiation therapy worked, check for other signs of cancer, look for late side effects, and talk with you about your treatment and care. Your doctor or nurse will:

- **Examine you and review how you have been feeling.** Your doctor or nurse practitioner can prescribe medicine or suggest other ways to treat any side effects you may have.

- **Order lab and imaging tests.** These may include blood tests, x-rays, or CT, MRI, or PET scans.

- **Discuss treatment.** Your doctor or nurse practitioner may suggest that you have more treatment, such as extra radiation treatments, chemotherapy, or both.

- **Answer your questions and respond to your concerns.** It may be helpful to write down your questions ahead of time and bring them with you. You can find sample questions on pages 51 and 52.

After radiation therapy is over, what symptoms should I look for?

You have gone through a lot with cancer and radiation therapy. Now you may be even more aware of your body and how you feel each day. Pay attention to changes in your body and let your doctor or nurse know if you have:

- A pain that does not go away

- New lumps, bumps, swellings, rashes, bruises, or bleeding

- Appetite changes, **nausea**, **vomiting**, diarrhea, or constipation

- Weight loss that you cannot explain

- A fever, cough, or hoarseness that does not go away

- Any other symptoms that worry you

See "Resources for Learning More" on page 59 for ways to learn more about radiation therapy.

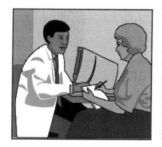

Make a list of questions and problems you want to discuss with your doctor or nurse. Be sure to bring this list to your follow-up visits. See pages 51 and 52 for sample questions.

www.cancer.gov

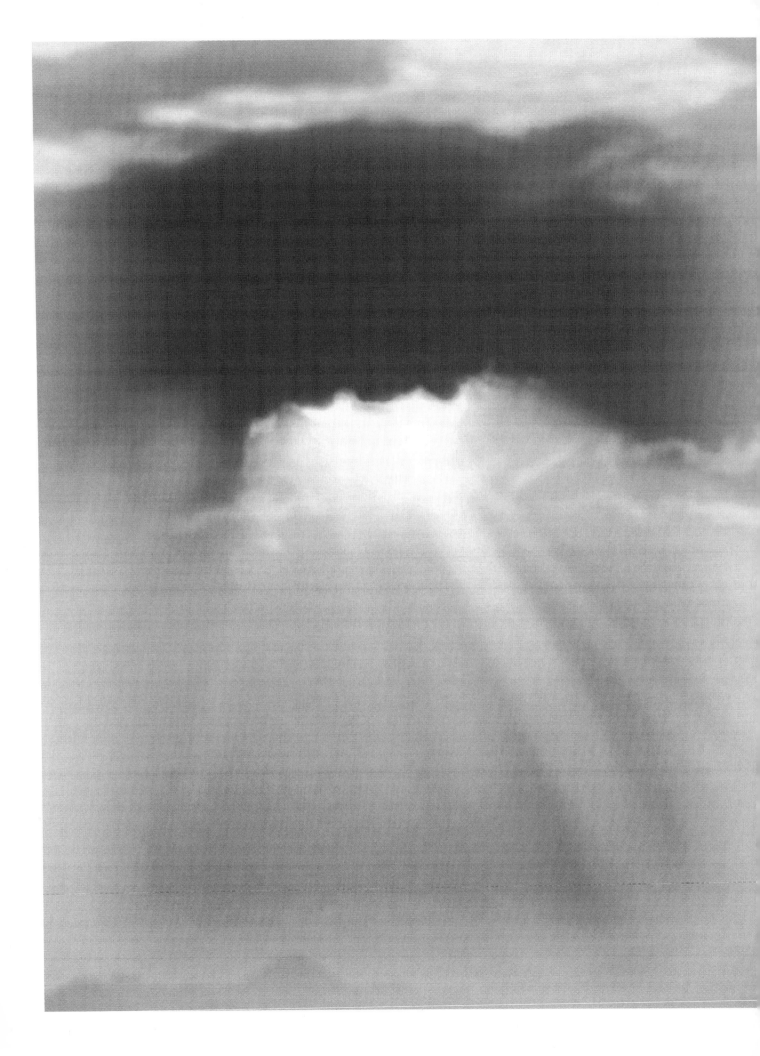

External Beam Radiation Therapy

What is external beam radiation therapy?

External beam radiation therapy comes from a machine that aims radiation at your cancer. The machine is large and may be noisy. It does not touch you, but rotates around you, sending radiation to your body from many directions.

External beam radiation therapy is a **local treatment**, meaning that the radiation is aimed only at a specific part of your body. For example, if you have lung cancer, you will get radiation to your chest only and not the rest of your body.

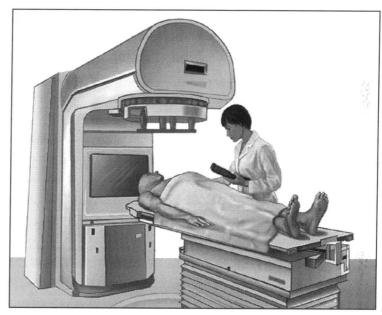

External beam radiation therapy comes from a machine that aims radiation at your cancer.

How often will I get external beam radiation therapy?

Most people get external beam radiation therapy once a day, 5 days a week, Monday through Friday. Treatment lasts for 2 to 10 weeks, depending on the type of cancer you have and the goal of your treatment. The time between your first and last radiation therapy sessions is called a course of treatment.

Radiation is sometimes given in smaller doses twice a day (**hyperfractionated radiation therapy**). Your doctor may prescribe this type of treatment if he or she feels that it will work better. Although side effects may be more severe, there may be fewer late side effects. Doctors are doing research to see which types of cancer are best treated this way.

www.cancer.gov

| **Where do I go for external beam radiation therapy?** | Most of the time, you will get external beam radiation therapy as an outpatient. This means that you will have treatment at a clinic or radiation therapy center and will not have to stay in the hospital. |

| **What happens before my first external beam radiation treatment?** | You will have a 1- to 2-hour meeting with your doctor or nurse before you begin radiation therapy. At this time, you will have a physical exam, talk about your medical history, and maybe have imaging tests. Your doctor or nurse will discuss external beam radiation therapy, its benefits and side effects, and ways you can care for yourself during and after treatment. You can then choose whether to have external beam radiation therapy. |

If you agree to have external beam radiation therapy, you will be scheduled for a treatment planning session called a **simulation**. At this time:

- A radiation oncologist and radiation therapist will define your treatment area (also called a **treatment port** or **treatment field**). This refers to the places in your body that will get radiation. You will be asked to lie very still while x-rays or scans are taken to define the treatment area.

- The radiation therapist will then put small marks (tattoos or dots of colored ink) on your skin to mark the treatment area. You will need these marks throughout the course of radiation therapy. The radiation therapist will use them each day to make sure you are in the correct position. Tattoos are about the size of a freckle and will remain on your skin for the rest of your life. Ink markings will fade over time. Be careful not to remove them and make sure to tell the radiation therapist if they fade or lose color.

> *Tell your radiation therapist if your ink marks begin to fade or lose color.*

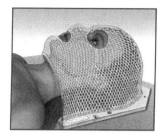

If you are getting radiation to the head, you may need a mask.

- You may need a body mold. This is a plastic or plaster form that helps keep you from moving during treatment. It also helps make sure that you are in the exact same position each day of treatment.

- If you are getting radiation to the head, you may need a mask. The mask has air holes, and holes can be cut for your eyes, nose, and mouth. It attaches to the table where you will lie to receive your treatments. The mask helps keep your head from moving so that you are in the exact same position for each treatment.

If the body mold or mask makes you feel anxious, see page 13 for ways to relax during treatment.

What should I wear when I get external beam radiation therapy?

Wear clothes that are comfortable and made of soft fabric, such as cotton. Choose clothes that are easy to take off, since you may need to change into a hospital gown or show the area that is being treated. Do not wear clothes that are tight, such as close-fitting collars or waistbands, near your treatment area. Also, do not wear jewelry, BAND-AIDS®, powder, lotion, or deodorant in or near your treatment area, and do not use deodorant soap before your treatment.

What happens during treatment sessions?

- You may be asked to change into a hospital gown or robe.

- You will go to a treatment room where you will receive radiation.

- Depending on where your cancer is, you will either sit in a chair or lie down on a treatment table. The radiation therapist will use your body mold and skin marks to help you get into position.

- You may see colored lights pointed at your skin marks. These lights are harmless and help the therapist position you for treatment each day.

- You will need to stay very still so the radiation goes to the exact same place each time. You can breathe as you always do and do not have to hold your breath.

The radiation therapist will leave the room just before your treatment begins. He or she will go to a nearby room to control the radiation machine and watch you on a TV screen or through a window. You are not alone, even though it may feel that way. The radiation therapist can see you on the screen or through the window. He or she can hear and talk with you through a speaker in your treatment room. Make sure to tell the therapist if you feel sick or are uncomfortable. He or she can stop the radiation machine at any time. You cannot feel, hear, see, or smell radiation.

Your entire visit may last from 30 minutes to 1 hour. Most of that time is spent setting you in the correct position. You will get radiation for only 1 to 5 minutes. If you are getting IMRT, your treatment may last longer. Your visit may also take longer if your treatment team needs to take and review x-rays.

> *Your radiation therapist can see, hear, and talk with you at all times while you are getting external beam radiation therapy.*

Will external beam radiation therapy make me radioactive?	No, external beam radiation therapy does not make people radioactive. You may safely be around other people, even babies and young children.

How can I relax during my treatment sessions?

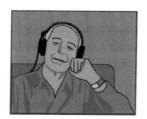

- Bring something to read or do while in the waiting room.
- Ask if you can listen to music or books on tape.
- Meditate, breathe deeply, use imagery, or find other ways to relax. To learn more about ways to relax, see *Facing Forward: Life After Cancer Treatment*, a book from the National Cancer Institute. You can order a free copy at http://www.cancer.gov/publications or 1-800-4-CANCER.

For ways to learn more about external beam radiation therapy, see the Resources for Learning More on page 59.

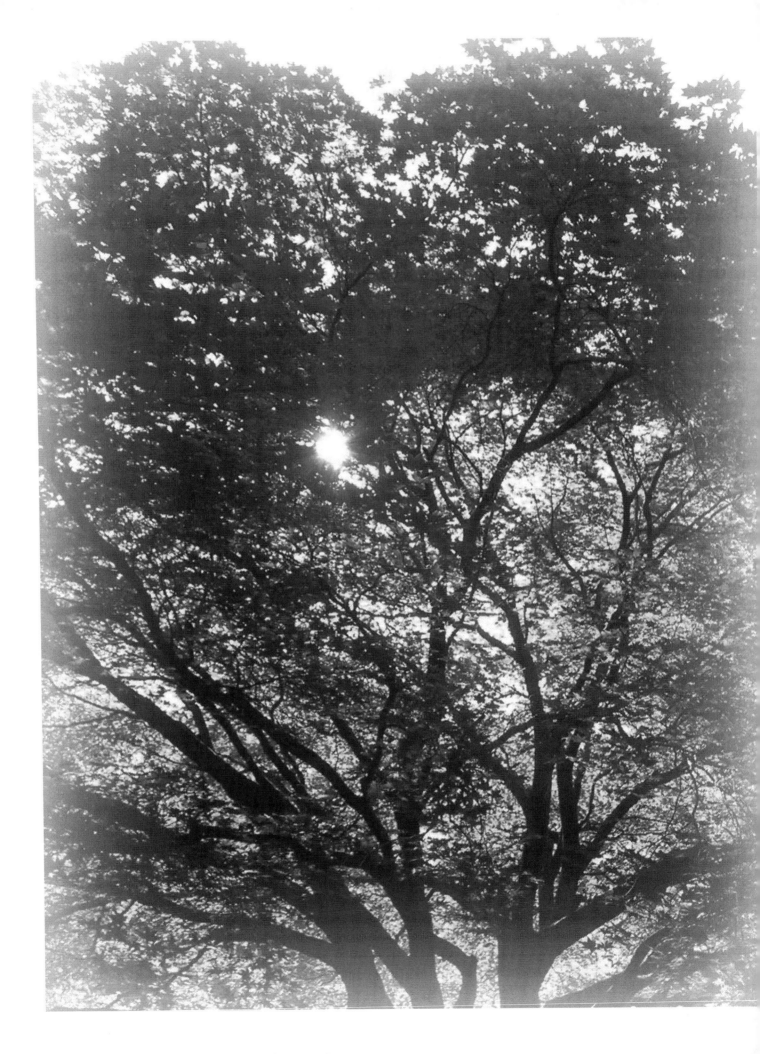

Internal Radiation Therapy

What is internal radiation therapy?

Internal radiation therapy is a form of treatment where a source of radiation is put inside your body. One form of internal radiation therapy is called **brachytherapy**. In brachytherapy, the radiation source is a solid in the form of seeds, ribbons, or capsules, which are placed in your body in or near the cancer cells. This allows treatment with a high dose of radiation to a smaller part of your body. Internal radiation can also be in a liquid form. You receive liquid radiation by drinking it, by swallowing a pill, or through an IV. Liquid radiation travels throughout your body, seeking out and killing cancer cells.

Brachytherapy may be used with people who have cancers of the head, neck, breast, uterus, cervix, prostate, gall bladder, esophagus, eye, and lung. Liquid forms of internal radiation are most often used with people who have thyroid cancer or non-Hodgkin's lymphoma. You may also get internal radiation along with other types of treatment, including external beam radiation, chemotherapy, or surgery.

What happens before my first internal radiation treatment?

You will have a 1- to 2-hour meeting with your doctor or nurse before you begin internal radiation therapy. At this time, you will have a physical exam, talk about your medical history, and maybe have imaging tests. Your doctor will discuss the type of internal radiation therapy that is best for you, its benefits and side effects, and ways you can care for yourself during and after treatment. You can then choose whether to have internal radiation therapy.

How is brachytherapy put in place?

Most brachytherapy is put in place through a **catheter**, which is a small, stretchy tube. Sometimes, it is put in place through a larger device called an **applicator**. When you decide to have brachytherapy, your doctor will place the catheter or applicator into the part of your body that will be treated.

What happens when the catheter or applicator is put in place?

You will most likely be in the hospital when your catheter or applicator is put in place. Here is what to expect:

- You will either be put to sleep or the area where the catheter or applicator goes will be numbed. This will help prevent pain when it is put in.

- Your doctor will place the catheter or applicator in your body.

- If you are awake, you may be asked to lie very still while the catheter or applicator is put in place. If you feel any discomfort, tell your doctor or nurse so he or she can give you medicine to help manage the pain.

> *Tell your doctor or nurse if you are in pain.*

What happens after the catheter or applicator is placed in my body?

Once your treatment plan is complete, radiation will be placed inside the catheter or applicator. The radiation source may be kept in place for a few minutes, many days, or the rest of your life. How long the radiation is in place depends on which type of brachytherapy you get, your type of cancer, where the cancer is in your body, your health, and other cancer treatments you have had.

What are the types of brachytherapy?

There are three types of brachytherapy:

- **Low-dose rate (LDR) implants.** In this type of brachytherapy, radiation stays in place for 1 to 7 days. You are likely to be in the hospital during this time. Once your treatment is finished, your doctor will remove the radiation sources and your catheter or applicator.

- **High-dose rate (HDR) implants.** In this type of brachytherapy, the radiation source is in place for 10 to 20 minutes at a time and then taken out. You may have treatment twice a day for 2 to 5 days or once a week for 2 to 5 weeks. The schedule depends on your type of cancer. During the course of treatment, your catheter or applicator may stay in place, or it may be put in place before each treatment. You may be in the hospital during this time, or you may make daily trips to the hospital to have the radiation source put in place. Like LDR implants, your doctor will remove your catheter or applicator once you have finished treatment.

- **Permanent implants.** After the radiation source is put in place, the catheter is removed. The implants always stay in your body, while the radiation gets weaker each day. You may need to limit your time around other people when the radiation is first put in place. Be extra careful not to spend time with children or pregnant women. As time goes by, almost all the radiation will go away, even though the implant stays in your body.

What happens while the radiation is in place?

- Your body will give off radiation once the radiation source is in place. With brachytherapy, your body fluids (urine, sweat, and saliva) will not give off radiation. With liquid radiation, your body fluids will give off radiation for a while.

- Your doctor or nurse will talk with you about safety measures that you need to take.

- If the radiation you receive is a very high dose, safety measures may include:
  - Staying in a private hospital room to protect others from radiation coming from your body
  - Being treated quickly by nurses and other hospital staff. They will provide all the care you need, but they may stand at a distance and talk with you from the doorway to your room.

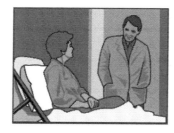

- Your visitors will also need to follow safety measures, which may include:
  - Not being allowed to visit when the radiation is first put in
  - Needing to check with the hospital staff before they go to your room
  - Keeping visits short (30 minutes or less each day). The length of visits depends on the type of radiation being used and the part of your body being treated.
  - Standing by the doorway rather than going into your hospital room
  - Not having visits from children younger than 18 and pregnant women

You may also need to follow safety measures once you leave the hospital, such as not spending much time with other people. Your doctor or nurse will talk with you about the safety measures you should follow when you go home.

What happens when the catheter is taken out after treatment with LDR or HDR implants?

- You will get medicine for pain before the catheter or applicator is removed.

- The area where the catheter or applicator was might be tender for a few months.

- There is no radiation in your body after the catheter or applicator is removed. It is safe for people to be near you—even young children and pregnant women.

- For 1 to 2 weeks, you may need to limit activities that take a lot of effort. Ask your doctor what kinds of activities are safe for you.

For ways to learn more about internal radiation therapy, see Resources for Learning More on page 59.

Your Feelings During Radiation Therapy

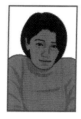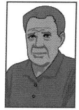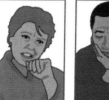

At some point during radiation therapy, you may feel:

- Anxious
- Depressed
- Afraid
- Angry
- Frustrated
- Helpless
- Alone

Having cancer and going through treatment is stressful.

It is normal to have these kinds of feelings. Living with cancer and going through treatment is stressful. You may also feel **fatigue**, which can make it harder to cope with these feelings.

How can I cope with my feelings during radiation therapy?

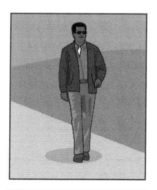

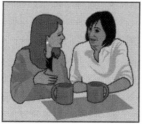

There are many things you can do to cope with your feelings during treatment. Here are some things that have worked for other people:

- **Relax and meditate.** You might try thinking of yourself in a favorite place, breathing slowly while paying attention to each breath, or listening to soothing music. These kinds of activities can help you feel calmer and less stressed.

- **Exercise.** Many people find that light exercise (such as walking, biking, yoga, or water aerobics) helps them feel better. Talk with your doctor or nurse about types of exercise that you can do.

- **Talk with others.** Talk about your feelings with someone you trust. You may choose a close friend, family member, chaplain, nurse, social worker, or psychologist. You may also find it helpful to talk to someone else who is going through radiation therapy.

- **Join a support group.** Cancer **support groups** are meetings for people with cancer. These groups allow you to meet others facing the same problems. You will have a

www.cancer.gov

chance to talk about your feelings and listen to other people talk about theirs. You can learn how others cope with cancer, radiation therapy, and side effects. Your doctor, nurse, or social worker can tell you about support groups near where you live. Some support groups also meet over the Internet, which can be helpful if you cannot travel or find a meeting in your area.

- ■ **Talk to your doctor or nurse about things that worry or upset you.** You may want to ask about seeing a counselor. Your doctor may also suggest that you take medicine if you find it very hard to cope with these feelings.

Ways to Learn More

To learn more about ways to cope with your feelings, read *Taking Time: Support for People with Cancer*, a book from the National Cancer Institute. You can get a free copy at http://www.cancer.gov/publications or 1-800-4-CANCER (1-800-422-6237).

CancerCare, Inc.

Offers free support, information, financial assistance, and practical help to people with cancer and their loved ones.

Toll-free: 1-800-813-HOPE (1-800-813-4673)

E-mail: info@cancercare.org

Online: http://www.cancercare.org

The Wellness Community

Provides free psychological and emotional support to people with cancer and their families.

Toll-free: 1-888-793-WELL (1-888-793-9355)

Phone: 202-659-9709

Online: http://www.thewellnesscommunity.org

E-mail: help@thewellnesscommunity.org

Radiation Therapy Side Effects

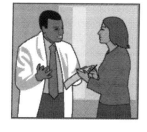

Side effects are problems that can happen as a result of treatment. They may happen with radiation therapy because the high doses of radiation used to kill cancer cells can also damage healthy cells in the treatment area. Side effects are different for each person. Some people have many side effects; others have hardly any. Side effects may be more severe if you also receive chemotherapy before, during, or after your radiation therapy.

Talk to your radiation therapy team about your chances of having side effects. The team will watch you closely and ask if you notice any problems. If you do have side effects or other problems, your doctor or nurse will talk with you about ways to manage them.

Common Side Effects

Many people who get radiation therapy have skin changes and some fatigue. Other side effects depend on the part of your body being treated.

Skin changes may include dryness, itching, peeling, or blistering. These changes occur because radiation therapy damages healthy skin cells in the treatment area. You will need to take special care of your skin during radiation therapy. To learn more, see page 40.

Fatigue is often described as feeling worn out or exhausted. There are many ways to manage fatigue. To learn more, see page 26.

Depending on the part of your body being treated, you may also have:

- Diarrhea
- Hair loss in treatment area
- Mouth problems
- Nausea and vomiting
- Sexual changes
- Swelling
- Trouble swallowing
- Urinary and bladder changes

Most of these side effects go away within 2 months after radiation therapy is finished.

Late side effects may first occur 6 or more months after radiation therapy is over. They vary by the part of your body that was treated and the dose of radiation you received. Late side effects may include **infertility**, joint problems, lymphedema, mouth problems, and secondary cancer. Everyone is different, so talk to your doctor or nurse about whether you might have late side effects and what signs to look for. See page 47 for more information on late side effects.

Radiation Therapy Side Effects and Ways To Manage Them, starting on page 24, explains each side effect in more detail and includes ways you and your doctor or nurse can help manage them.

Radiation Therapy Side Effects At-A-Glance

Radiation therapy side effects depend on the part of your body being treated. You can use the chart on page 23 to see which side effects might affect you. Find the part of your body being treated in the column on the left, then read across the row to see the side effects. A checkmark means that you may get this side effect. Ask your doctor or nurse about your chances of getting each side effect.

To learn more about each side effect, see the page listed in the top row of the table on page 23.

> *Talk to your radiation therapy team about your chances of getting side effects. Show them the chart on the next page.*

Radiation Therapy Side Effects At-A-Glance

- Find the part of your body being treated in the column on the left.
- Read across the row.
- A checkmark means you may get the side effect listed.

	Diarrhea (See page 24)	Fatigue (See page 26)	Hair Loss (on the part of the body being treated) (See page 28)	Mouth Changes (See page 30)	Nausea and Vomiting (See page 34)	Sexual and Fertility Changes (See page 36)	Skin Changes (See page 40)	Throat Changes (See page 43)	Urinary and Bladder Changes (See page 45)	Other Side Effects
Brain		✔	✔		✔		✔			Headache, Blurry vision
Breast		✔	✔				✔			Tenderness, Swelling
Chest		✔	✔				✔	✔		Cough, Shortness of breath
Head and Neck		✔	✔	✔			✔	✔		Earaches, Taste changes
Pelvic Area	✔	✔	✔		✔	✔	✔		✔	
Rectum	✔	✔	✔			✔	✔		✔	
Stomach and Abdomen	✔	✔	✔		✔		✔		✔	

Diarrhea

What it is

Diarrhea is frequent bowel movements which may be soft, formed, loose, or watery. Diarrhea can occur at any time during radiation therapy.

Why it occurs

Radiation therapy to the pelvis, stomach, and abdomen can cause diarrhea. People get diarrhea because radiation harms the healthy cells in the large and small bowels. These areas are very sensitive to the amount of radiation needed to treat cancer.

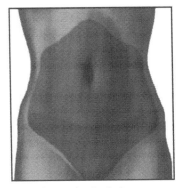

Radiation to the shaded area may cause diarrhea.

Ways to manage

When you have diarrhea:

- **Drink 8 to 12 cups of clear liquid per day.** See page 53 for ideas of drinks and foods that are clear liquids.

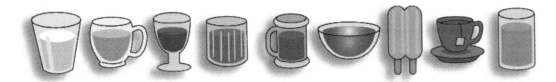

  If you drink liquids that are high in sugar (such as fruit juice, sweet iced tea, Kool-Aid®, or Hi-C®) ask your nurse or dietitian if you should mix them with water.

- **Eat many small meals and snacks.** For instance, eat 5 or 6 small meals and snacks rather than 3 large meals.

- **Eat foods that are easy on the stomach (which means foods that are low in fiber, fat, and lactose).** See page 55 for other ideas of foods that are easy on the stomach. If your diarrhea is severe, your doctor or nurse may suggest the BRAT diet, which stands for bananas, rice, applesauce, and toast.

- **Take care of your rectal area.** Instead of toilet paper, use a baby wipe or squirt of water from a spray bottle to clean yourself after bowel movements. Also, ask your nurse about taking **sitz baths,** which is a warm-water bath taken in a sitting position that covers only the hips and buttocks. Be sure to tell your doctor or nurse if your rectal area gets sore.

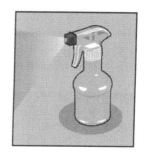

- **Stay away from:**
    - Milk and dairy foods, such as ice cream, sour cream, and cheese
    - Spicy foods, such as hot sauce, salsa, chili, and curry dishes
    - Foods or drinks with caffeine, such as regular coffee, black tea, soda, and chocolate
    - Foods or drinks that cause gas, such as cooked dried beans, cabbage, broccoli, soy milk, and other soy products
    - Foods that are high in fiber, such as raw fruits and vegetables, cooked dried beans, and whole wheat breads and cereals
    - Fried or greasy foods
    - Food from fast food restaurants

- **Talk to your doctor or nurse.** Tell them if you are having diarrhea. He or she will suggest ways to manage it. He or she may also suggest taking medicine, such as Imodium®.

To learn more about dealing with diarrhea during cancer treatment, see *Eating Hints: Before, During, and After Cancer Treatment*, a book from the National Cancer Institute. You can get a free copy at http://www.cancer.gov/publications or 1-800-4-CANCER (1-800-422-6237).

Fatigue

What it is

Fatigue from radiation therapy can range from a mild to an extreme feeling of being tired. Many people describe fatigue as feeling weak, weary, worn out, heavy, or slow.

Why it occurs

Fatigue can happen for many reasons. These include:

- **Anemia**
- Anxiety
- Depression
- Infection
- Lack of activity
- Medicines

> Fatigue is a common side effect, and there is a good chance that you will feel some level of fatigue from radiation therapy.

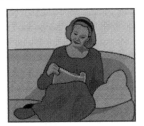

Fatigue can also come from the effort of going to radiation therapy each day or from stress. Most of the time, you will not know why you feel fatigue.

How long it lasts

When you first feel fatigue depends on a few factors, which include your age, health, level of activity, and how you felt before radiation therapy started.

Fatigue can last from 6 weeks to 12 months after your last radiation therapy session. Some people may always feel fatigue and, even after radiation therapy is over, will not have as much energy as they did before.

Ways to manage

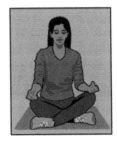

- **Try to sleep at least 8 hours each night.** This may be more sleep than you needed before radiation therapy. One way to sleep better at night is to be active during the day. For example, you could go for walks, do yoga, or ride a bike. Another way to sleep better at night is to relax before going to bed. You might read a book, work on a jigsaw puzzle, listen to music, or do other calming hobbies.

- **Plan time to rest.** You may need to nap during the day. Many people say that it helps to rest for just 10 to 15 minutes. If you do nap, try to sleep for less than 1 hour at a time.

- **Try not to do too much.** With fatigue, you may not have enough energy to do all the things you want to do. Stay active, but choose the activities that are most important to you. For example, you might go to work but not do housework, or watch your children's sports events but not go out to dinner.

- **Exercise.** Most people feel better when they get some exercise each day. Go for a 15- to 30-minute walk or do stretches or yoga. Talk with your doctor or nurse about how much exercise you can do while having radiation therapy.

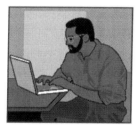

- **Plan a work schedule that is right for you.** Fatigue may affect the amount of energy you have for your job. You may feel well enough to work your full schedule, or you may need to work less—maybe just a few hours a day or a few days each week. You may want to talk with your boss about ways to work from home so you do not have to commute. And you may want to think about going on medical leave while you have radiation therapy.

- **Plan a radiation therapy schedule that makes sense for you.** You may want to schedule your radiation therapy around your work or family schedule. For example, you might want to have radiation therapy in the morning so you can go to work in the afternoon.

- **Let others help you at home.** Check with your insurance company to see whether it covers home care services. You can also ask family members and friends to help when you feel fatigue. Home care staff, family members, and friends can assist with household chores, running errands, or driving you to and from radiation therapy visits. They might also help by cooking meals for you to eat now or freeze for later.

- **Learn from others who have cancer.** People who have cancer can help each other by sharing ways to manage fatigue. One way to meet other people with cancer is by joining a support group—either in person or online. Talk with your doctor or nurse to learn more about support groups.

- **Talk with your doctor or nurse.** If you have trouble dealing with fatigue, your doctor may prescribe medicine (called **psychostimulants**) that can help decrease fatigue, give you a sense of well-being, and increase your appetite. Your doctor may also suggest treatments if you have anemia, depression, or are not able to sleep at night.

Hair Loss

What it is
Hair loss (also called **alopecia**) is when some or all of your hair falls out.

> You will lose hair only on the part of your body being treated.

Why it occurs
Radiation therapy can cause hair loss because it damages cells that grow quickly, such as those in your hair roots.

Hair loss from radiation therapy only happens on the part of your body being treated. This is not the same as hair loss from chemotherapy, which happens all over your body. For instance, you may lose some or all of the hair on your head when you get radiation to your brain. But if you get radiation to your hip, you may lose pubic hair (between your legs) but not the hair on your head.

How long it lasts
You may start losing hair in your treatment area 2 to 3 weeks after your first radiation therapy session. It takes about a week for all the hair in your treatment area to fall out. Your hair may grow back 3 to 6 months after treatment is over. Sometimes, though, the dose of radiation is so high that your hair never grows back.

Once your hair starts to grow back, it may not look or feel the way it did before. Your hair may be thinner, or curly instead of straight. Or it may be darker or lighter in color than it was before.

Ways to manage hair loss on your head

Before hair loss:

- **Decide whether to cut your hair or shave your head.** You may feel more in control of hair loss when you plan ahead. Use an electric razor to prevent nicking yourself if you decide to shave your head.

- **If you plan to buy a wig, do so while you still have hair.** The best time to select your wig is before radiation therapy begins or soon after it starts. This way, the wig will match the color and style of your own hair. Some people take their wig to their hair stylist. You will want to have your wig fitted once you have lost your hair. Make sure to choose a wig that feels comfortable and does not hurt your scalp.

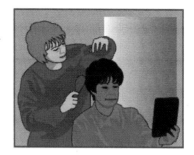

- **Check with your health insurance company to see whether it will pay for your wig.** If it does not, you can deduct the cost of your wig as a medical expense on your income taxes. Some groups also sponsor free wig banks. Ask your doctor, nurse, or social worker if he or she can refer you to a free wig bank in your area.

- **Be gentle when you wash your hair.** Use a mild shampoo, such as a baby shampoo. Dry your hair by patting (not rubbing) it with a soft towel.

- **Do not use curling irons, electric hair dryers, curlers, hair bands, clips, or hair sprays.** These can hurt your scalp or cause early hair loss.

- **Do not use products that are harsh on your hair.** These include hair colors, perms, gels, mousse, oil, grease, or pomade.

After hair loss:

- **Protect your scalp.** Your scalp may feel tender after hair loss. Cover your head with a hat, turban, or scarf when you are outside. Try not to be in places where the temperature is very cold or very hot. This means staying away from the direct sun, sun lamps, and very cold air.

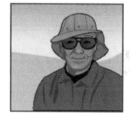

- **Stay warm.** Your hair helps keep you warm, so you may feel colder once you lose it. You can stay warmer by wearing a hat, turban, scarf, or wig.

Ways to learn more

American Cancer Society

Offers a variety of services to people with cancer and their families, including referrals to low-cost wig banks.

Toll-free: 1-800-ACS-2345 (1-800-227-2345)
Phone: 404-320-3333
Online: http://www.cancer.org

Mouth Changes

What they are

Radiation therapy to the head or neck can cause problems such as:

- Mouth sores (little cuts or ulcers in your mouth)
- Dry mouth (also called **xerostomia**) and throat
- Loss of taste
- Tooth decay
- Changes in taste (such as a metallic taste when you eat meat)
- Infections of your gums, teeth, or tongue
- Jaw stiffness and bone changes
- Thick, rope-like saliva

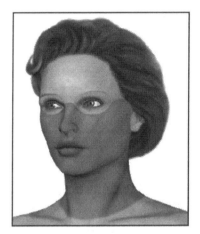

Radiation to the shaded area may cause mouth changes.

Why they occur

Radiation therapy kills cancer cells and can also damage healthy cells such as those in the glands that make saliva and the soft, moist lining of your mouth.

How long they last

Some problems, like mouth sores, may go away after treatment ends. Others, such as taste changes, may last for months or even years. Some problems, like dry mouth, may never go away.

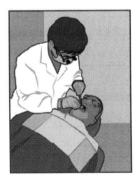

Visit a dentist at least 2 weeks before starting radiation therapy to your head or neck.

Ways to manage

- If you are getting radiation therapy to your head or neck, **visit a dentist at least 2 weeks before treatment starts.** At this time, your dentist will examine your teeth and mouth and do any needed dental work to make sure your mouth is as healthy as possible before radiation therapy. If you cannot get to the dentist before treatment starts, ask your doctor if you should schedule a visit soon after treatment begins.

- **Check your mouth every day.** This way, you can see or feel problems as soon as they start. Problems can include mouth sores, white patches, or infection.

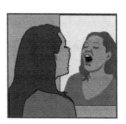

- **Keep your mouth moist.** You can do this by:
  - Sipping water often during the day
  - Sucking on ice chips
  - Chewing sugar-free gum or sucking on sugar-free hard candy
  - Using a saliva substitute to help moisten your mouth
  - Asking your doctor to prescribe medicine that helps increase saliva

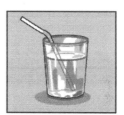
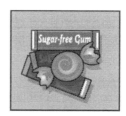

- **Clean your mouth, teeth, gums, and tongue.**
  - Brush your teeth, gums, and tongue after every meal and at bedtime.
  - Use an extra-soft toothbrush. You can make the bristles softer by running warm water over them just before you brush.
  - Use a fluoride toothpaste.
  - Use a special fluoride gel that your dentist can prescribe.
  - Do not use mouthwashes that contain alcohol.
  - Gently floss your teeth every day. If your gums bleed or hurt, avoid those areas but floss your other teeth.
  - Rinse your mouth every 1 to 2 hours with a solution of 1/4 teaspoon baking soda and 1/8 teaspoon salt mixed in 1 cup of warm water.
  - If you have dentures, make sure they fit well and limit how long you wear them each day. If you lose weight, your dentist may need to adjust them.
  - Keep your dentures clean by soaking or brushing them each day.

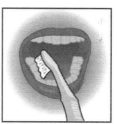
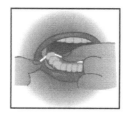
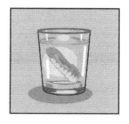

- **Be careful what you eat when your mouth is sore.**
  - Choose foods that are easy to chew and swallow.
  - Take small bites, chew slowly, and sip liquids with your meals.
  - Eat moist, soft foods such as cooked cereals, mashed potatoes, and scrambled eggs.
  - Wet and soften food with gravy, sauce, broth, yogurt, or other liquids.
  - Eat foods that are warm or at room temperature.

- **Stay away from things that can hurt, scrape, or burn your mouth, such as:**
  - Sharp, crunchy foods such as potato or corn chips
  - Hot foods
  - Spicy foods such as hot sauce, curry dishes, salsa, and chili
  - Fruits and juices that are high in acid such as tomatoes, oranges, lemons, and grapefruits
  - Toothpicks or other sharp objects
  - All tobacco products, including cigarettes, pipes, cigars, and chewing tobacco
  - Drinks that contain alcohol

Do not use tobacco or drink alcohol while you are getting radiation therapy to your head or neck.

- **Stay away from foods and drinks that are high in sugar.** Foods and drinks that have a lot sugar (such as regular soda, gum, and candy) can cause tooth decay.

- **Exercise your jaw muscles.**
  Open and close your mouth 20 times as far as you can without causing pain. Do this exercise 3 times a day, even if your jaw isn't stiff.

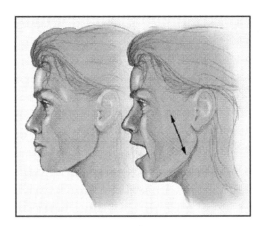

Exercise your jaw 3 times a day.

- **Medicine.** Ask your doctor or nurse about medicines that can protect your saliva glands and the moist tissues that line your mouth.

- **Call your doctor or nurse when your mouth hurts.** There are medicines and other products, such as mouth gels, that can help control mouth pain.

- **You will need to take extra good care of your mouth for the rest of your life.** Ask your dentist how often you will need dental check-ups and how best to take care of your teeth and mouth after radiation therapy is over.

Ways to learn more

National Oral Health Information Clearinghouse

A service of the National Institute of Dental and Craniofacial Research that provides oral health information for special care patients.

Phone: 301-402-7364
Online: http://www.nidcr.nih.gov

Smokefree.gov

Provides resources, including information on quit lines, a step-by-step cessation guide, and publications, to help you or someone you care about quit smoking.

Toll-free: 1-877-44U-QUIT (1-877-448-7848)
Online: http://www.smokefree.gov

Nausea and Vomiting

What they are

Radiation therapy can cause nausea, vomiting, or both. Nausea is when you feel sick to your stomach and feel like you are going to throw up. Vomiting is when you throw up food and fluids. You may also have **dry heaves**, which happen when your body tries to vomit even though your stomach is empty.

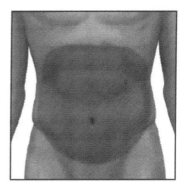

Radiation to the shaded area may cause nausea and vomiting.

Why they occur

Nausea and vomiting can occur after radiation therapy to the stomach, small intestine, colon, or parts of the brain. Your risk for nausea and vomiting depends on how much radiation you are getting, how much of your body is in the treatment area, and whether you are also having chemotherapy.

How long they last

Nausea and vomiting may occur 30 minutes to many hours after your radiation therapy session ends. You are likely to feel better on days that you do not have radiation therapy.

Ways to manage

- **Prevent nausea.** The best way to keep from vomiting is to prevent nausea. One way to do this is by having bland, easy-to-digest foods and drinks that do not upset your stomach. These include toast, gelatin, and apple juice. To learn more, see the list of foods and drinks that are easy on the stomach on page 55.

- **Try to relax before treatment.** You may feel less nausea if you relax before each radiation therapy treatment. You can do this by spending time doing activities you enjoy, such as reading a book, listening to music, or other hobbies.

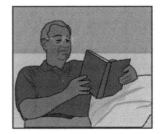

- **Plan when to eat and drink.** Some people feel better when they eat before radiation therapy; others do not. Learn the best time for you to eat and drink. For example, you might want a snack of crackers and apple juice 1 to 2 hours before radiation therapy. Or, you might feel better if you have treatment on an empty stomach, which means not eating 2 to 3 hours before treatment.

- **Eat small meals and snacks.** Instead of eating 3 large meals each day, you may want to eat 5 or 6 small meals and snacks. Make sure to eat slowly and do not rush.

> Eat 5 or 6 small meals and snacks each day instead of 3 large meals.

- **Have foods and drinks that are warm or cool (not hot or cold).** Before eating or drinking, let hot food and drinks cool down and cold food and drinks warm up.

- **Talk with your doctor or nurse.** He or she may suggest a special diet of foods to eat or prescribe medicine to help prevent nausea, which you can take 1 hour before each radiation therapy session. You might also ask your doctor or nurse about **acupuncture**, which may help relieve nausea and vomiting caused by cancer treatment.

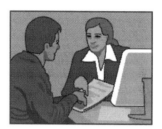

To learn more about dealing with nausea and vomiting during cancer treatment, see *Eating Hints: Before, During, and After Cancer Treatment*, a book from the National Cancer Institute. You can get a free copy at http://www.cancer.gov/publications or 1-800-4-CANCER (1-800-422-6237).

Sexual and Fertility Changes

What they are

Radiation therapy sometimes causes sexual changes, which can include hormone changes and loss of interest in or ability to have sex. It can also affect fertility during and after radiation therapy. For a woman, this means that she might not be able to get pregnant and have a baby. For a man, this means that he might not be able to get a woman pregnant. Sexual and fertility changes differ for men and women.

> Be sure to tell your doctor if you are pregnant before you start radiation therapy.

Problems for women include:

- Pain or discomfort when having sex
- Vaginal itching, burning, dryness, or atrophy (when the muscles in the vagina become weak and the walls of the vagina become thin)
- **Vaginal stenosis**, when the vagina becomes less elastic, narrows, and gets shorter
- Symptoms of menopause for women not yet in menopause. These include hot flashes, vaginal dryness, and not having your period.
- Not being able to get pregnant after radiation therapy is over

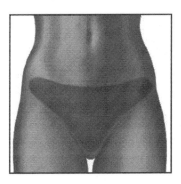

Radiation to the shaded area may cause sexual and fertility changes.

Problems for men include:

- **Impotence** (also called **erectile dysfunction** or ED), which means not being able to have or keep an erection
- Not being able to get a woman pregnant after radiation therapy is over due to fewer or less effective sperm

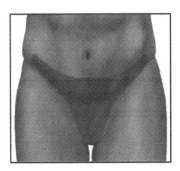

Why they occur

Sexual and fertility changes can happen when people get radiation therapy to the pelvic area. For women, this includes radiation to the vagina, uterus, or ovaries. For men, this includes radiation to the testicles or prostate. Many sexual side effects are caused by scar tissue from radiation therapy. Other problems, such as fatigue, pain, anxiety, or depression, can affect your interest in having sex.

How long they last

After radiation therapy is over, most people want to have sex as much as they did before treatment. Many sexual side effects go away after treatment ends. But you may have problems with hormone changes and fertility for the rest of your life. If you are able to get pregnant or father a child after you have finished radiation therapy, it should not affect the health of the baby.

Ways to manage

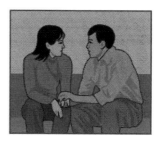

For both men and women, it is important to be open and honest with your spouse or partner about your feelings, concerns, and how you prefer to be intimate while you are getting radiation therapy.

For women, here are some issues to discuss with your doctor or nurse:

- **Fertility.** Before radiation therapy starts, let your doctor or nurse know if you think you might want to get pregnant after your treatment ends. He or she can talk with you about ways to preserve your fertility, such as preserving your eggs to use in the future.

- **Sexual problems.** You may or may not have sexual problems. Your doctor or nurse can tell you about side effects you can expect and suggest ways for coping with them.

- **Birth control.** It is very important that you do not get pregnant while having radiation therapy. Radiation therapy can hurt the fetus at all stages of pregnancy. If you have not yet gone through menopause, talk with your doctor or nurse about birth control and ways to keep from getting pregnant.

- **Pregnancy.** Make sure to tell your doctor or nurse if you are already pregnant.

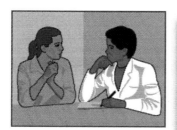

Talk to your doctor or nurse if you want to have children in the future.

- **Stretching your vagina.** Vaginal stenosis is a common problem for women who have radiation therapy to the pelvis. This can make it painful to have sex. You can help by stretching your vagina using a **dilator** (a device that gently stretches the tissues of the vagina). Ask your doctor or nurse where to find a dilator and how to use it.

- **Lubrication.** Use a special lotion for your vagina (such as Replens®) once a day to keep it moist. When you have sex, use a water- or mineral oil-based lubricant (such as K-Y Jelly® or Astroglide®).

- **Sex.** Ask your doctor or nurse whether it is okay for you to have sex during radiation therapy. Most women can have sex, but it is a good idea to ask and be sure. If sex is painful due to vaginal dryness, you can use a water- or mineral oil-based lubricant.

For men, here are some issues to discuss with your doctor or nurse:

- **Fertility.** Before you start radiation therapy, let your doctor or nurse know if you think you might want to father children in the future. He or she may talk with you about ways to preserve your fertility before treatment starts, such as banking your sperm. Your sperm will need to be collected before you begin radiation therapy.

- **Impotence.** Your doctor or nurse can let you know whether you are likely to become impotent and how long it might last. Your doctor can prescribe medicine or other treatments that may help.

- **Sex.** Ask if it is okay for you to have sex during radiation therapy. Most men can have sex, but it is a good idea to ask and be sure.

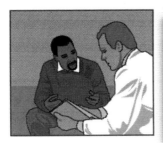

If you want to father children in the future, your sperm will need to be collected before you begin treatment.

Ways to learn more

American Cancer Society

Offers a variety of services to patients and their families. It also supports research, provides printed materials, and conducts educational programs.

Toll-free: 1-800-ACS-2345 (1-800-227-2345)
Phone: 404-320-3333
Online: http://www.cancer.org

fertileHope

Dedicated to helping people with cancer faced with infertility.

Toll-free: 1-888-994-HOPE (1-888-994-4673)
Online: http://www.fertilehope.org

Skin Changes

What they are

Radiation therapy can cause skin changes in your treatment area. Here are some common skin changes:

- **Redness.** Your skin in the treatment area may look as if you have a mild to severe sunburn or tan. This can occur on any part of your body where you are getting radiation.

- **Pruritus.** The skin in your treatment area may itch so much that you always feel like scratching. This causes problems because scratching too much can lead to **skin breakdown** and infection.

- **Dry and peeling skin.** This is when the skin in your treatment area gets very dry—much drier than normal. In fact, your skin may be so dry that it peels like it does after a sunburn.

- **Moist reaction.** Radiation kills skin cells in your treatment area, causing your skin to peel off faster than it can grow back. When this happens, you can get sores or ulcers. The skin in your treatment area can also become wet, sore, or infected. This is more common where you have skin folds, such as your buttocks, behind your ears, under your breasts. It may also occur where your skin is very thin, such as your neck.

- **Swollen skin.** The skin in your treatment area may be swollen and puffy.

Why they occur

Radiation therapy causes skin cells to break down and die. When people get radiation almost every day, their skin cells do not have enough time to grow back between treatments. Skin changes can happen on any part of the body that gets radiation.

How long they last

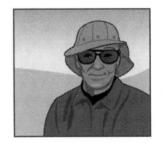

Skin changes may start a few weeks after you begin radiation therapy. Many of these changes often go away a few weeks after treatment is over. But even after radiation therapy ends, you may still have skin changes. Your treated skin may always look darker and blotchy. It may feel very dry or thicker than before. And you may always burn quickly and be sensitive to the sun. You will always be at risk for skin cancer in the treatment area. Be sure to avoid tanning beds and protect yourself from the sun by wearing a hat, long sleeves, long pants, and sunscreen with an SPF of 30 or higher.

Ways to manage

- **Skin care.** Take extra good care of your skin during radiation therapy. Be gentle and do not rub, scrub, or scratch in the treatment area. Also, use creams that your doctor prescribes.

> *Take extra good care of your skin during radiation therapy. Be gentle and do not rub, scrub, or scratch.*

- **Do not put anything on your skin that is very hot or cold.** This means not using heating pads, ice packs, or other hot or cold items on the treatment area. It also means washing with lukewarm water.

- **Be gentle when you shower or take a bath.** You can take a lukewarm shower every day. If you prefer to take a lukewarm bath, do so only every other day and soak for less than 30 minutes. Whether you take a shower or bath, make sure to use a mild soap that does not have fragrance or deodorant in it. Dry yourself with a soft towel by patting, not rubbing, your skin. Be careful not to wash off the ink markings that you need for radiation therapy.

> *Be careful not to wash off the ink markings you need for radiation therapy.*

- **Use only those lotions and skin products that your doctor or nurse suggests.** If you are using a prescribed cream for a skin problem or acne, you must tell your doctor or nurse before you begin radiation treatment. Check with your doctor or nurse before using any of the following skin products:

  - Bubble bath
  - Cornstarch
  - Cream
  - Deodorant
  - Hair removers
  - Makeup
  - Oil
  - Ointment
  - Perfume
  - Powder
  - Soap
  - Sunscreen

- **Cool, humid places.** Your skin may feel much better when you are in cool, humid places. You can make rooms more humid by putting a bowl of water on the radiator or using a humidifier. If you use a humidifier, be sure to follow the directions about cleaning it to prevent bacteria.

- **Soft fabrics.** Wear clothes and use bed sheets that are soft, such as those made from cotton.

- **Do not wear clothes that are tight and do not breathe,** such as girdles and pantyhose.

- **Protect your skin from the sun every day.** The sun can burn you even on cloudy days or when you are outside for just a few minutes. Do not go to the beach or sun bathe. Wear a broad-brimmed hat, long-sleeved shirt, and long pants when you are outside. Talk with your doctor or nurse about sunscreen lotions. He or she may suggest that you use a sunscreen with an SPF of 30 or higher. You will need to protect your skin from the sun even after radiation therapy is over, since you will have an increased risk of skin cancer for the rest of your life.

- **Do not use tanning beds.** Tanning beds expose you to the same harmful effects as the sun.

- **Adhesive tape.** Do not put bandages, BAND-AIDS®, or other types of sticky tape on your skin in the treatment area. Talk with your doctor or nurse about ways to bandage without tape.

- **Shaving.** Ask your doctor or nurse if you can shave the treated area. If you can shave, use an electric razor and do not use pre-shave lotion.

- **Rectal area.** If you have radiation therapy to the rectal area, you are likely to have skin problems. These problems are often worse after a bowel movement. Clean yourself with a baby wipe or squirt of water from a spray bottle. Also ask your nurse about sitz baths (a warm-water bath taken in a sitting position that covers only the hips and buttocks.)

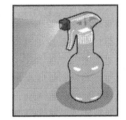

- **Talk with your doctor or nurse.** Some skin changes can be very serious. Your treatment team will check for skin changes each time you have radiation therapy. Make sure to report any skin changes that you notice.

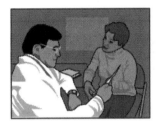

- **Medicine.** Medicines can help with some skin changes. They include lotions for dry or itchy skin, antibiotics to treat infection, and other drugs to reduce swelling or itching.

Throat Changes

What they are

Radiation therapy to the neck or chest can cause the lining of your throat to become inflamed and sore. This is called **esophagitis**. You may feel as if you have a lump in your throat or burning in your chest or throat. You may also have trouble swallowing.

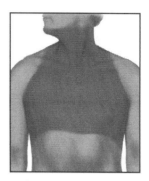

Radiation to the shaded area may cause throat changes.

Why they occur

Radiation therapy to the neck or chest can cause throat changes because it not only kills cancer cells, but can also damage the healthy cells that line your throat. Your risk for throat changes depends on how much radiation you are getting, whether you are also having chemotherapy, and whether you use tobacco and alcohol while you are getting radiation therapy.

How long they last

You may notice throat changes 2 to 3 weeks after starting radiation. You will most likely feel better 4 to 6 weeks after radiation therapy has finished.

Ways to manage

- **Be careful what you eat when your throat is sore.**
  - Choose foods that are easy to swallow.
  - Cut, blend, or shred foods to make them easier to eat.
  - Eat moist, soft foods such as cooked cereals, mashed potatoes, and scrambled eggs.
  - Wet and soften food with gravy, sauce, broth, yogurt, or other liquids.
  - Drink cool drinks.
  - Sip drinks through a straw.
  - Eat foods that are cool or at room temperature.

- **Eat small meals and snacks.** It may be easier to eat a small amount of food at one time. Instead of eating 3 large meals each day, you may want to eat 5 or 6 small meals and snacks.

- **Choose foods and drinks that are high in calories and protein.** When it hurts to swallow, you may eat less and lose weight. It is important to keep your weight the same during radiation therapy. Having foods and drinks that are high in calories and protein can help you. See the chart of foods and drinks that are high in calories and protein on page 54 for ideas.

- **Sit upright and bend your head slightly forward when you are eating or drinking.** Remain sitting or standing upright for at least 30 minutes after eating.

- **Don't have things that can burn or scrape your throat, such as:**
  - Hot foods and drinks
  - Spicy foods
  - Foods and juices that are high in acid, such as tomatoes and oranges
  - Sharp, crunchy foods such as potato or corn chips
  - All tobacco products, such as cigarettes, pipes, cigars, and chewing tobacco
  - Drinks that contain alcohol

- **Talk with a dietitian.** He or she can help make sure you eat enough to maintain your weight. This may include choosing foods that are high in calories and protein and foods that are easy to swallow.

- **Talk with your doctor or nurse.** Let your doctor or nurse know if you notice throat changes, such as trouble swallowing, feeling as if you are choking, or coughing while eating or drinking. Also, let him or her know if you have pain or lose any weight. Your doctor can prescribe medicines that may help relieve your symptoms, such as antacids, gels that coat your throat, and pain killers.

> *Let your doctor or nurse know if you:*
> - *Have trouble swallowing*
> - *Feel as if you are choking*
> - *Cough while you are eating or drinking*

Ways to learn more

To learn more about dealing with throat problems, the following books from the National Cancer Institute may help you: *Eating Hints: Before, During, and After Cancer Treatment* and *Pain Control: Support for People With Cancer.* You can get free copies at www.cancer.gov/publications or by calling 1-800-4-CANCER (1-800-422-6237).

Smokefree.gov

Provides resources, including information on quit lines, a step-by-step cessation guide, and publications, to help you or someone you care about quit smoking.

Toll-free: 1-877-44U-QUIT (1-877-448-7848)
Online: http://www.smokefree.gov

Urinary and Bladder Changes

What they are

Radiation therapy can cause urinary and bladder problems, which can include:

- Burning or pain when you begin to **urinate** or after you empty your bladder

- Trouble starting to urinate

- Trouble emptying your bladder

- Frequent, urgent need to urinate

- **Cystitis,** a swelling (**inflammation**) in your urinary tract

- **Incontinence,** when you cannot control the flow of urine from your bladder, especially when coughing or sneezing

- Frequent need to get up during sleep to urinate

- Blood in your urine

- Bladder spasms, which are like painful muscle cramps

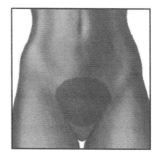

Radiation to the shaded area may cause urinary and bladder changes.

Why they occur

Urinary and bladder problems may occur when people get radiation therapy to the prostate or bladder. Radiation therapy can harm the healthy cells of the bladder wall and urinary tract, which can cause inflammation, ulcers, and infection.

How long they last

Urinary and bladder problems often start 3 to 5 weeks after radiation therapy begins. Most problems go away 2 to 8 weeks after treatment is over.

Drink 6 to 8 cups of fluids each day.

Ways to manage

- **Drink a lot of fluids.** This means 6 to 8 cups of fluids each day. Drink enough fluids so that your urine is clear to light yellow in color.

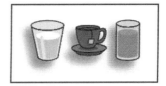

- **Avoid coffee, black tea, alcohol, spices, and all tobacco products.**

- **Talk with your doctor or nurse if you think you have urinary or bladder problems.** He or she may ask for a urine sample to make sure that you do not have an infection.

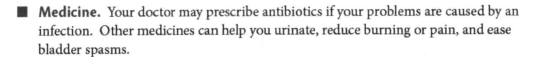

- **Talk to your doctor or nurse if you have incontinence.** He or she may refer you to a physical therapist who will assess your problem. The therapist can give you exercises to improve bladder control.

- **Medicine.** Your doctor may prescribe antibiotics if your problems are caused by an infection. Other medicines can help you urinate, reduce burning or pain, and ease bladder spasms.

Late Side Effects

Late side effects are those that first occur at least 6 months after radiation therapy is over. Late side effects are rare, but they do happen. It is important to have follow-up care with a radiation oncologist or nurse practitioner for the rest of your life.

Whether you get late side effects will depend on:

- The part of your body that was treated
- The dose and length of your radiation therapy
- If you received chemotherapy before, during, or after radiation therapy

Your doctor or nurse will talk with you about late side effects and discuss ways to help prevent them, symptoms to look for, and how to treat them if they occur.

Some late side effects are brain problems, infertility, joint problems, **lymphedema**, mouth problems, and secondary cancers.

Brain Changes

What they are

Radiation therapy to the brain can cause problems months or years after treatment ends. Side effects can include memory loss, problems doing math, movement problems, incontinence, trouble thinking, or personality changes. Sometimes, dead tumor cells can form a mass in the brain, which is called **radiation necrosis**.

Ways to manage

You will need to have check-ups with your doctor or nurse for the rest of your life. If you have symptoms, you will have tests to see whether they are due to the cancer or late side effects.

If you have late side effects, your doctor or nurse practitioner:

- Will talk with you about ways to manage late side effects
- May refer you to a physical, occupational, or speech therapist who can help with problems caused by late side effects
- May prescribe medicine or suggest surgery to help with the symptoms

Late Radiation Therapy Side Effects and Ways to Manage Them

Infertility

What it is

For men, infertility means not being able to get a woman pregnant. For women, it means not being able to get pregnant.

Ways men with infertility can become a parent:

- **Donor sperm.** This means getting a woman pregnant with sperm given by another man.
- **Adoption.** Taking on legal responsibility for someone else's child and raising the child as your own.

Ways women with infertility can become a parent:

- **Donor embryos.** Another couple donates a fertilized egg that your doctor implants in your uterus to carry until birth.
- **Donor eggs.** An egg (donated by someone else) is fertilized by your partner's sperm. Your doctor implants the fertilized egg in your uterus to carry until birth.
- **Surrogacy.** Another woman carries and gives birth to your child. She can also donate her egg, which is fertilized by your partner's sperm.
- **Adoption.** Taking on legal responsibility for someone else's child and raising the child as your own.

Joint Changes

What they are

Radiation therapy can cause scar tissue and weakness in the part of the body that was treated. This can lead to loss of motion in your joints, such as your jaw, shoulders, or hips. Joint problems can show up months or years after radiation therapy is over.

Ways to manage

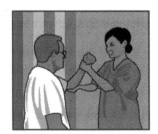

Notice early signs of joint problems. These signs include:

- Trouble getting your mouth to open wide
- Pain when you make certain movements, such as reaching over your head or putting your hand in a back pocket

Talk with your doctor or nurse. He or she may refer you to a physical therapist who will assess your joint problems. The therapist can give you exercises to decrease pain, increase strength, and improve movement.

Late Radiation Therapy Side Effects and Ways to Manage Them

Lymphedema

What it is

Swelling in an arm or a leg caused by a build up of lymph fluid. Lymphedema can happen if your lymph nodes were removed during surgery or damaged by radiation therapy.

Tell your doctor or nurse if you notice swelling in the arm or leg on the side where you had radiation.

Ways to manage

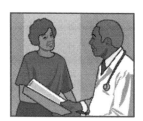

- **Meet with your doctor or nurse.** Ask about your risk of lymphedema and ways to prevent it. Your doctor or nurse may suggest exercises, medicines, or compression garments (special wraps to put on your legs or arms). You might also want to ask for a referral to a physical therapist.

- **Be active.** Exercise can help prevent and treat lymphedema. Ask your doctor, nurse, or physical therapist which exercises are safe for you to do.

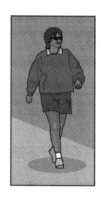

- **Take care of your arm or leg.**
    - Use skin lotion at least once a day.
    - Avoid sunburn. Use sunscreen with an SPF of 30 or higher and wear long sleeves and long pants if you need to be in the sun.
    - Wear gloves when you garden or cook.
    - Clip your toenails straight across, file your fingernails, and do not cut your cuticles.
    - Keep your feet clean and wear dry, cotton socks.
    - Clean cuts with soap and water and then use antibacterial ointment.
    - Avoid extreme hot or cold, such as ice packs or heating pads.
    - Do not put pressure on your arm or leg. For example, do not cross your legs when sitting or carry your purse on the side that had radiation.
    - Wear loose clothes that do not have tight elastic cuffs or waistbands.

- **Notice early signs of lymphedema.** Let your doctor or nurse know if you have:
    - Pain or a sense of heaviness in your arm or leg
    - A feeling of tightness in your arm or leg
    - Trouble putting on your shoes or rings
    - Weakness in your arm or leg
    - Redness, swelling, or other signs of infection

www.cancer.gov

Mouth Changes

What they are

Radiation therapy to your head and neck can cause late side effects in your mouth. Problems may include dry mouth, cavities, or bone loss in the jaw.

Ways to manage

- **Visit your dentist.** You may be asked to have your teeth checked every 1 to 2 months for at least 6 months after radiation treatment ends. During this time, your dentist will look for changes in your mouth, teeth, and jaw.

- **Exercise your jaw.** Open and close your mouth 20 times as far as you can without causing pain. Do this exercise 3 times a day, even if your jaw isn't stiff.

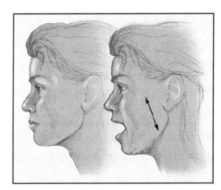

Exercise your jaw 3 times a day.

- **Take good care of your teeth and gums.** This means flossing, using daily fluoride treatments, and brushing your teeth after meals and before you go to bed.

- **Have your dentist contact your radiation oncologist before you have dental or gum surgery.** This includes not having teeth pulled from the part of your mouth that received radiation. There may be other options than surgery.

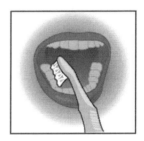

Secondary Cancer

What it is

Radiation therapy can cause a new cancer many years after you have finished treatment. This does not happen very often.

Ways to manage

You will need to have check-ups with your radiation oncologist or nurse practitioner for the rest of your life to check for cancer—the one you were treated for and any new cancer that may occur.

See Resources for Learning More on pages 59 and 60 for ways to learn more about late side effects.

Questions To Ask Your Doctor or Nurse

Here are some questions you might want to ask your doctor or nurse. You may want to write down their answers so you can review them again later.

What kind of radiation therapy will I get?

_____

_____

How can radiation therapy help?

_____

_____

How many weeks will my course of radiation therapy last?

_____

_____

What kinds of side effects should I expect during my course of radiation therapy?

_____

_____

Will these side effects go away after radiation therapy is over?

_____

_____

What kind of late side effects should I expect after radiation therapy is over?

_____

_____

What can I do to manage these side effects?
_____
_____

What will you do to manage these side effects?
_____
_____

How can I learn more about radiation therapy?
_____
_____

Which sections should I read in this book?
_____
_____

Lists of Foods and Liquids

Clear Liquids

This list may help if you have diarrhea. See page 24 for more information.

Types of Liquids	Includes...
Soups	Bouillon Clear, fat-free broth Consommé Strained vegetable broth
Drinks	Apple juice Clear carbonated beverages Cranberry or grape juice Fruit-flavored drinks Fruit punch Sports drinks Tea Water
Sweets	Fruit ices without fruit pieces Fruit ices without milk Honey Jelly Plain gelatin dessert Popsicles

Foods and Drinks That Are High in Calories or Protein

This list may help if you need ideas for keeping your weight the same. See pages 5 and 43 for more information.

Types of Foods and Drinks	Includes . . .
Soups	Cream soups
Drinks	Instant breakfast shakes Milkshakes Whole milk (instead of low-fat or skim)
Main meals and other foods	Beans, legumes Butter, margarine, or oil Cheese Chicken, fish, or beef Cottage cheese Cream cheese on crackers or celery Deviled ham Eggs, such as scrambled or deviled eggs Muffins Nuts, seeds, wheat germ Peanut butter
Desserts and other sweets	Custards Frozen yogurt Ice cream Puddings Yogurt
Replacements and other supplements	Powdered milk added to foods (pudding, milkshakes, or scrambled eggs) High-protein supplements, such as Ensure® and Carnation® Instant Breakfast®

Foods and Drinks That Are Easy on the Stomach

This list may help if you have diarrhea or nausea and vomiting. See pages 24 and 34 for more information.

Types of Foods and Drinks	Includes . . .
Soups	Clear broth, such as chicken or beef
Drinks	Clear carbonated beverages
	Cranberry or grape juice
	Fruit-flavored drinks
	Fruit punch
	Sports drinks
	Tea
	Water
Main meals and snacks	Boiled potatoes
	Chicken, broiled or baked without the skin
	Crackers
	Cream of wheat
	Noodles
	Oatmeal
	Pretzels
	Rice
	Toast
Sweets	Angel food cake
	Canned peaches
	Gelatin
	Sherbet
	Yogurt

Words To Know

3-D conformal radiation therapy (ray-dee-AY-shun): Uses a computer to create a 3-D picture of a cancer tumor. This allows doctors to give the highest possible dose of radiation to the tumor, while sparing the normal tissue as much as possible.

Acupuncture (AK-yoo-PUNK-cher): A technique of inserting thin needles through the skin at specific points on the body to control pain and side effects. It is a type of complementary and alternative medicine.

Alopecia (al-oh-PEE-shuh): Hair loss; when some or all of your hair falls out.

Anemia (a-NEE-mee-a): A problem in which the number of red blood cells is below normal.

Applicator: A large device used to place brachytherapy in the body.

Brachytherapy (BRAKE-ee-THER-a-pee): Treatment in which a solid radioactive substance is implanted inside your body, near or next to the cancer cells.

CT scan: A series of detailed pictures of areas inside the body, taken from different angles; the pictures are created by a computer linked to an x-ray machine.

Catheter: A flexible tube used to place brachytherapy in the body.

Course of treatment: All of your radiation therapy sessions.

Cystitis: Inflammation in your urinary tract.

Diet: Foods you eat (does not always refer to a way to lose weight).

Dilator (DYE-lay-tor): A device that gently stretches the tissues of the vagina.

Dry heaves: A problem that occurs when your body tries to vomit even though your stomach is empty.

Erectile dysfunction (e-WRECK-tile dis-FUNK-shun): Not able to have an erection of the penis adequate for sexual intercourse. Also called impotence.

Esophagitis: Inflammation of the esophagus (the tube that carries food from the mouth to the stomach).

External beam radiation therapy (ray-dee-AY-shun): Treatment in which a radiation source from outside your body aims radiation at your cancer cells.

Fatigue: A feeling of being weary or exhausted.

Follow-up care: Check-up appointments that you have after your course of radiation therapy is over.

Hyperfractionated radiation therapy ((hy-per-FRAK-shuh-NAYT-id ray-dee-AY-shun THAYR-uh-pee): Treatment in which radiation is given in smaller doses twice a day.

Imaging tests: Tests that produce pictures of areas inside the body.

Implant: Radioactive material put in your body through a sealed thin wire, catheter, or tube.

Impotence (IM-po-tense): Not able to have an erection of the penis adequate for sexual intercourse. Also called erectile dysfunction.

IMRT (intensity-modulated radiation therapy): A technique that uses a computer to deliver precise radiation doses to a cancer tumor or specific areas within the tumor.

Incontinence (in-KAHN-tih-nens): A problem in which you cannot control the flow of urine from your bladder.

Infertility: Not being able to produce children.

Inflammation: Redness, swelling, pain, and/or a feeling of heat in an area of the body.

Internal radiation therapy (ray-dee-AY-shun): Treatment in which a radioactive substance is put inside your body.

Intraoperative radiation (ray-dee-AY-shun): Radiation treatment aimed directly at cancer during surgery.

Late side effects: Side effects that first occur 6 or more months after radiation therapy is finished.

Local treatment: Radiation is aimed at only the part of your body with cancer.

Lymphedema: A problem in which excess fluid collects in tissue and causes swelling. It may occur in the arm or leg after lymph vessels or lymph nodes in the underarm or groin are removed by surgery or treated with radiation.

Medical leave: Taking time off work for a while due to a medical problem.

MRI (magnetic resonance imaging): A procedure in which radio waves and a powerful magnet linked to a computer are used to create detailed pictures of areas inside the body.

Nausea: When you have an upset stomach or queasy feeling and feel like you are going to throw up.

Pelvis: The area between your legs. Also called the groin.

Permanent implants: Radioactive pellets or seeds that always stay in your body.

PET (Positron emission tomography) scan: A procedure in which a small amount of radioactive glucose (sugar) is injected into a vein, and a scanner is used to make detailed, computerized pictures of areas inside the body where the glucose is used. Because cancer cells often use more glucose than normal cells, the pictures can be used to find cancer cells in the body.

Pruritus: Severe itching.

Psychostimulants: Medicines that can help decrease fatigue, give a sense of well-being, and increase appetite.

Radiation necrosis: A problem in which dead tumor cells form a mass in the brain.

Radiation oncologist (ray-dee-AY-shun on-KO-lo-jist): A doctor who specializes in using radiation to treat cancer.

Radiation therapy (ray-dee-AY-shun): High doses of radiation used to treat cancer and other diseases.

Radiotherapy (RAY-dee-o-THER-a-pee): Another word for radiation therapy.

Simulation (sim-you-LAY-shun): A process used to plan radiation therapy so that the target area is precisely located and marked.

Sitz bath: A warm-water bath taken in a sitting position that covers only the hips and buttocks.

Skin breakdown: A side effect from radiation therapy in which the skin in the treatment area peels off faster than it can grow back.

Support groups: Meetings for people who share the same problems, such as cancer.

Treatment field: One or more places on your body where the radiation will be aimed. Also called treatment port.

Treatment port: One or more places on your body where the radiation will be aimed. Also called treatment field.

Urinate (YOOR-in-nate): Emptying your bladder of urine.

Vaginal stenosis (ste-NO-sis): A problem in which the vagina narrows and gets smaller.

Vomiting: When you get sick and throw up your food.

Xerostomia: Dry mouth.

Resources for Learning More

National Cancer Institute

Cancer Information Service

Answers questions about cancer clinical trials and cancer-related services and helps users find information on the NCI Web site. Provides NCI printed materials.

Toll-free: 1-800-4-CANCER (1-800-422-6237)
TTY: 1-800-332-8615
Online: http://www.cancer.gov
Chat online: http://www.cancer.gov/help

American Cancer Society

Offers a variety of services to patients and their families. It also supports research, provides printed materials, and conducts educational programs.

Toll-free: 1-800-ACS-2345 (1-800-227-2345)
Online: http://www.cancer.org

American Society for Therapeutic Radiology and Oncology

A society of radiation oncology professionals who specialize in treating patients with radiation therapy. Patients can get information on treating cancer with radiation and find a radiation oncologist in their area.

Toll-free: 1-800-962-7876
Online: http://www.astro.org

CancerCare, Inc.

Offers free support, information, financial assistance, and practical help to people with cancer and their loved ones.

Toll-free: 1-800-813-HOPE (1-800-813-4673)
Online: http://www.cancercare.org
E-mail: info@cancercare.org

fertileHOPE

Dedicated to helping people with cancer faced with infertility.

Toll-free: 1-888-994-HOPE (1-888-994-4673)
Online: http://www.fertilehope.org

National Brain Tumor Foundation

Dedicated to providing information and support for brain tumor patients, their family members, and health care professionals, while supporting innovative research into better treatment options and a cure for brain tumors.

Toll-free: 1-800-934-2873
Online: http://www.braintumor.org

National Lymphedema Network

Provides education and guidance to lymphedema patients, health care professionals, and the general public by disseminating information on the prevention and management of primary and secondary lymphedema.

Toll-free: 800-541-3259
Phone: 510-208-3200
Online: http://www.lymphnet.org
E-mail: nln@lymphnet.org

National Oral Health Information Clearinghouse

A service of the National Institute of Dental and Craniofacial Research that provides oral health information for special care patients.

Phone: 301-402-7364
Online: http://www.nidcr.nih.gov

The Wellness Community

Provides free psychological and emotional support to cancer patients and their loved ones.

Toll-free: 1-888-793-WELL (1-888-793-9355)
Phone: 202-659-9709
Online: http://www.thewellnesscommunity.org
E-mail: help@thewellnesscommunity.org

Made in the USA
Middletown, DE
09 July 2018